THE HIDDEN SECRETS *of* FOODS AND HERBS

By Johnny Brown

© 2023 Johnny Brown.

All rights reserved.

No part of this publication may be reproduced, distributed, or transmitted in any form or by any means, including photocopying, recording, or other electronic or mechanical methods, without the prior written permission of the publisher, except in the case of brief quotations embodied in critical reviews and certain other noncommercial uses permitted by copyright law.

Any unauthorized usage of the materials contained within this publication is a violation of applicable laws, subject to penalties under copyright infringement.

Edited by Deborah Brown

Formatted and Designed by Katherine Peters

Table of Contents

PART ONE: HEALING FROM WITHIN

Cancer and the Alkalinity of the Body 8
High Blood Pressure 12
The Benefits of Rest/Sleep 14
Lung Inflammation 15
The Secret of Fasting 17

PART TWO: THE HIDDEN SECRET OF FOOD AND HERBS

Garlic 21
Ginger 21
Turmeric 22
Kale 23
Blueberry 24
Blackberries 25
Raspberries 26
Strawberries 27
Beet Root 27
Pomegranate 29
Clove 30
Brussels Sprout 32

Cabbage 33

Broccoli 33

Yam 35

Dasheen 35

Papaya 36

Avocado 39

Pineapple 42

Soursop Fruit 43

Jackfruit 44

Breadfruit 46

Strong Back 47

Jamaican-Spanish Needle 48

Periwinkle 49

Lantana Camara 51

Stinging Nettle 52

PART THREE: CLEANSING THE BODY

Revitalizing Herb 55

Kalawalla 56

Sarsaparilla Root 57

Irish Moss [Sea Moss] 57

Granadilla Fruit 58

Mimosa Pudica 59

BIOGRAPHY

Growing up in Jamaica, folk remedies have always been a part of my life. Living with aging grandparents in the countryside taught you to appreciate the goodness of local herbs. As my grandfather, Pupa, often said, "Fever grass a di king of fevers, cerasee cure every bilious." I have grown up knowing and using simple herbal teas and tonics to treat any illness I may have had. I remember attending Sabbath services with my grandparents and learning how God healed His people from their sicknesses and diseases, and how all the fruits and herbs were given to man as food; I was fascinated.

Unfortunately, growing up with aging poor grandparents never gave me the opportunity for formal education; however, it has always been my dream to become a healer one day, using just the plants that God prepared for us to be our food and healer.

In 1962, when I was ten years old, I left the care of my grandparents to reside with my mother, Pearl Frankson, in Old Harbour, St. Catherine. There I met my oldest sister and my two brothers. My mother was a raster woman who loved the Bible. The Bible and the belt became my teacher from that moment. I learned to read the Bible, which I believe is the greatest literacy teacher. Learning to read strengthened my desire to become an herbal healer. My life was not an ideal one, and I can remember running away from home on many occasions, forced to sleep in old cars that were left parked, the open air with the grass as my bed as well as unfinished houses. I started hanging out with bad friends and getting into trouble constantly. I started developing the habit of cursing and slowly lost the respect for older people that was ingrained in me by my grandparents.

My dream to become an herbal doctor was the only constant thing with me. I had visions of herbs and the magic they may produce for older people, which prompted me to change. One day in 19 74, I took up the Bible again, my mom was pleased, and my eyes slowly opened to God's wonders again. It was like a gift that kept giving. I started making roots/tonics for the people around me. My first herbal book was *Back to Eden*, which taught me a lot about herbs. Since that day, herbs and natural plant foods have been my doctor, and I wish to share them with my brothers and sisters worldwide.

Johnny Brown.

PART ONE

HEALING FROM WITHIN

In the fast-paced and often chaotic world we live in, it's easy to overlook the incredible power that lies within our own bodies. We possess an innate ability to heal and restore ourselves, and this potential is amplified when we tap into the healing properties of nature. By nourishing our bodies with the right foods and harnessing the therapeutic benefits of herbs, we can unlock a profound journey of healing from within.

The concept of healing from within is rooted in the understanding that our bodies are designed to maintain equilibrium and thrive when provided with the right tools. Just as a garden flourishes when tended to with care, our bodies respond positively when we cultivate an environment conducive to healing.

At the core of this philosophy is recognizing that what we consume directly impacts our physical, mental, and emotional well-being. Every bite we take and every sip we drink has the potential to either nourish or harm our bodies. By choosing nutrient-dense foods and incorporating healing herbs into our diet, we can optimize our body's natural healing mechanisms.

This journey of healing from within is not limited to a single ailment or condition. It encompasses a holistic approach to well-being, addressing the root causes of various health concerns and promoting overall vitality. From chronic diseases to everyday ailments, the power of healing from within holds the potential to transform our lives.

Throughout this section, we will explore the remarkable impact that food and herbs can have on our health. We will delve into specific topics such as cancer and the alkalinity of the body, high blood pressure, the significance of rest and sleep, and the management of lung inflammation. By understanding the intricate relationship between nutrition, herbs, and disease, we will unveil the extraordinary potential of these natural remedies to restore balance and promote optimal health.

So, let us embark on this journey together as we embrace the profound wisdom of healing from within. By nourishing our bodies, supporting our immune systems, and cultivating a harmonious relationship with nature, we open the door to a life of vitality, resilience, and holistic well-being.

CANCER AND THE ALKALINITY OF THE BODY

Cancer is one of man's number one killers and is often incurable. Cancer is a generic term used to describe a large group of diseases that can affect any part of the body. It is often characterized as abnormal cell growth that rapidly multiplies and spreads within the body. Several signs portend cancer, such as;

- A significant and long-term change in our bowel and bladder habits. Lumps are found all around the body, most notably the breast.
- A sore that does not heal or unusual bleeding in the genital area, mouth, nose, throat, etc.
- A nagging cough, prolonged hoarseness, and difficulty swallowing are some of the most common signs of cancer.

Some of the common causes of cancer are due the smoking of tobacco, excessive alcohol consumption, unhealthy diet practices due to our lifestyle habits, obesity and lack of exercise as well as genetics and excessive exposure to UV rays.

To prevent cancer within the body or help eliminate cancer cells, how we treat our bodies must change. The very first thing I would like you to do is to have your body well alkaline in order to protect you from cancer. The reason to have the body well-alkaline is that cancer cannot survive in a well-alkaline system. Alkalinity helps with the body's PH balance, which is extremely important for normal functioning. The PH level balance for every living being (not only for cancer patients) is vital for overall health. Therefore, in order to get well and remain healthy, you need to maintain an alkaline environment in the body.

Cancer is a serious health risk that often leads to death and should never be taken lightly. Cancer can and may take many forms and all are killers. Some common forms of cancer are; breast cancer which more commonly affects women; however, men, to a lesser extent, are also affected by it as well. Another form of cancer that is associated with women's reproductive health is cervical and ovarian cancer.

Another form is lung cancer which is more common in men, although women are also at risk for developing this type of cancer. Lung cancer is rapidly approaching that same position for women and is often found in cigarette smokers.

If cancer is not treated in time and properly to completely eradicate it from the body, it will continue to spread and will eventually become fatal. Several steps must be taken when attempting to rid the body of cancer. The first step is to thoroughly cleanse the blood stream to remove toxins from the body. Removing toxins allows all the elimination organs, such as the skin, lungs, liver, kidney, and bowels to become active and remain active. Often, detoxing is done through herbal laxatives, which is a good way to cleanse the colon of any bad condition for optimal health. During the cleansing, changing the diet and switching to mostly fruit and vegetable diet is necessary. Beneficial fruits are those high in citrus and fiber, such as; oranges, grapefruit, lemon, cranberries, unsweetened blueberries, red raspberries, cherries, and pineapples. Other important fruits are avocado and tomato. The best fruits to eat are also those that have all ripened on the tree or vine.

Another thing of note when doing this cleansing is that tomatoes should be eaten separately from other fruits to be fully beneficial. This is important for the first ten days. Cleansing may last longer or shorter, depending on the condition of the patient. It is advisable not to mix citrus fruits together while using citrus juice.

Vegetable juice is very useful and important during cleansing as well. Green vegetables such as; celery, cucumber, parsley, lettuce, and other vegetables such as carrots may be consumed. However, mixing your fruits while making juices is not advisable; vegetables can be combined to create a very nutritious drink. There should be an equal balance of fruit and vegetable juices versus herbal tea mix per day in a 6:6 ratio—six glasses of juice and six glasses of herbal tea per day. If you are taking herbs as capsules, please ask the herbalist for the correct dose to avoid overdose. This is often followed by a glass of warm water (AS HOT AS CAN BE TAKEN COMFORTABLY). The herb must be taken 1 Hour before you take your juice.

While doing the cleansing, if there is significant weight loss after a few days, then it is advisable to switch from an all-juice diet and substitute juice for an alkaline nourishing vegetable soup/food.

Foods that promote an alkaline diet are green vegies, black rice, carrot, eggplant, olives, lima beans, onion, garlic, young beets, cornmeal, etc. A note of importance is that you should not simultaneously eat fruit/fruit juice with vegetable/vegetable juice. You should also be getting plenty of fresh air and exercise; allow yourself to soak up the sunshine in the early morning or evening. Good ventilation is necessary to cleanse the lungs and increase circulation. If the patient cannot go outside, you must avoid poorly lit areas and ensure that your environment is well-ventilated.

Taking a sweat bath is also beneficial to open up the pores of the skin, which will help to eliminate a lot of toxins through sweating. During the sweat bath, it is advisable to keep the head cool with a cold water rag or cloth. If the patient has heart issues, it is necessary to place an ice bag over the heart to increase circulation. Apply a hot and cold compress over the areas of the Stomach, Spleen, and Spine alternately. A thorough massage is also beneficial as this increases the blood flow around the body.

While cleansing the body does not cure cancer, it assists the body to be in an optimal condition to be healed. Some herbs that assist the body in eradicating cancer are RED CLOVER, BERDUCK ROOT, YELLOW DOCK ROOT, GOLDEN SEAL ROOT, GUM MERRH, ALOES, DANDELION ROOT, CHICK WEED, GUINEA HEN WEED, PAPAYA LEAF, SOUR SOP LEAF, Noni, and SMALL WILLOW FLOWER.

Here is a list of nourishing foods to eat during cancer treatment; Broccoli, Salmon, Brussels sprouts, Flax seed, Chia seed, Nuts, Avocado, Olive, Eggs, Peas and Beans, Blue berries, Swiss Chard, Water Melon, Olive oil, etc.

To allow the body to recover swiftly, the diet is extremely important and plays a crucial role. An unhealthy diet creates an acidic environment that greatly increases the risk of cancer and other health issues and provides cancer with the optimal environment to spread rapidly. There is a great saying that is a known truth, "FOR LIFE IS IN THE BLOOD." A healthy body means having a clean bloodstream free from all poisons and toxins, starting with a good diet.

A healthy body requires the following:

- Clean blood stream.
- A good diet.
- Healing herbs.
- Clean filtered water.
- Plenty of fresh air

- A good massage to increase blood flow.
- Plenty of sunshine.
- Exercise
- Good mental health.
- Plenty of Good Rest.

Often, we neglect these things, which is why we often get sick. However, we are reminded in God's words that he has provided us with the means to secure our health. GENESIS 1:29 states, "AND GOD SAID BEHOLD I HAVE GIVEN YOU EVERY HERB BEARING SEED WHICH IS UPON THE FACE OF ALL THE EARTH, AND EVERY TREE IN THE WHICH IS THE FRUIT OF A TREE YIELDING SEED TO YOU IT SHALL BE FOR MEAT AMEN." While we strive to practice good health, may the God of heaven and earth be with you and bless you with good health and long life.

HIGH BLOOD PRESSURE

In the case of eating an unbalanced diet, foods that have no life-giving properties and are rich in sodium content are one of the main causes of people having high blood pressure. Over-eating, especially unhealthy foods, is another major factor contributing to high blood pressure. This is one of the main reasons for obesity. The majority of persons diagnosed with this illness are often overweight, physically inactive, and often engage in a diet that has a high salt content.

Doctors and dieticians often advise limiting salt intake into the body so that the liver and kidneys will not be overburdened with an abundance of irritating foods.

People with high blood pressure frequently complain of frequent headaches, particularly in the morning, difficulty breathing, dizziness, flushed complexion, and blurred vision. This is because of a severe hypertensive crisis where the blood pressure has spiked more than 180/120mm hg. People who are often diagnosed with this condition may first be seen with heart failure or stroke symptoms. In fact, one of the most frequent causes of a stroke (cerebrovascular accident) or a heart attack (myocardial infraction) is hypertension.

To lower the sodium content within the blood, a high herbal enema should first be given to clean the waste matter within the colon. A dose of one teaspoon of Golden Seal in one pint of boiling water should be taken at least six times per day. Red Clover tea may be taken regularly and continuously because studies have shown that this herb can be used to purify the blood. In its unsweetened form, this tea may be used in place of 1/3 to half the required drinking water. These are a number of herbs that are very useful for high blood pressure. These are; Wild Cherry Bark, Hyssop, Vervain, Rue, Black and Blue cohosh. These herbs may be brewed into teas and integrated into the regular diet.

Once integrated into the regular diet, many herbs will improve overall health; however, sufficient rest is vital as it allows the body time to rejuvenate. Another thing to note is that a person suffering from high blood pressure should change their daily diet. Foods that should be avoided are bleached foods such as white flour sugar products. Other foods that should be excluded from the diet are red meats, coffee, mustard, alcohol and all forms of stimulating/energy products/drinks because they are very harmful. Tobacco smoking should also be excluded from your lifestyle practices as it is one of the main causes of a heart attack/stroke.

During colon cleansing, a fruit diet should be taken for the first 2-4 days. It is also highly recommended that the patient gets plenty of exercise, especially outdoor exercise, as exercising in the open allows for the practice of deep breathing exercises.

THE BENEFITS OF REST/SLEEP

We often find ourselves so busy with our daily lives and struggles that we often neglect a very important component of our health, rest. During consultations, one of the most frequent admissions is that patients suffering from high blood pressure are not getting enough rest. They are often bogged down and worried about their business affairs, or they have too many social duties that they fail to realize that they are not getting enough rest.

Sleep is very important to the normal functioning of the body. Sleep allows the brain to repair, re-energize and restore itself. I mention these things because, too often, we fail to realize that it is due to the body being overly tired that causes the blood pressure to rise abnormally. Rest is imperative to the body's normal functioning.

A warm bath at night and plenty of good sleep in a well-ventilated room will greatly lower your blood pressure. If you have trouble with sleeplessness, please take a herbal tea that will induce sleep. This tea is harmless and will leave no bad aftereffects. Following the above treatment and instructions will decrease your blood pressure and greatly aid your recovery. A hot and cold application to the spine, liver, spleen, and stomach and a cold towel rub in the morning upon rising will do great. A warm bath at night, a salt glow, and a hot and cold shower will also help. A general massage is excellent as it will aid in working the waste matter out of your system, equalizing the circulation and greatly relieving the heart and nerves. The blood pressure reflects the contractile power of your heart and the resistance of the blood vessels. Your blood pressure will increase slowly during your lifetime.

In other words, your normal blood pressure at age 30 is approximately 125, and at age 60, it is about 140 MM HG. This is what research shows that people who are weak physically have slightly lower blood pressure. Your blood pressure will rise to some degree during exercise, depending on the amount of exercise you are accustomed to. The more regularly you exercise, the less your blood pressure will rise. If your blood pressure is too high or too low, there may be something wrong with your arteries because your blood circulation is not going through. Therefore, a course of treatment must be given to improve the circulation. When this is done, it will help the blood pressure to return to normal.

There are two very important things that you can do to lower your blood pressure. Restrict the amount of salt in your diet and ensure you are not overweight. After using the above simple measures, if your blood pressure does not reduce to within the normal range, please see a medical doctor for more help to prevent a stroke or a heart attack. Coronary artery occlusion in people with high blood pressure requires water, garlic, coffee, fatty fish, beet root, cayenne pepper, apple, berries and dandelion. Please remember to keep an alkaline body for good health.

Genesis 1v 29 says, And God said, Behold, I have given you every herb bearing seed, which is upon the face of all the earth, and every tree, in the which is the fruit of a tree yielding seed; to you, it shall be for meat.

This is also your medicine, for your medicine is your food. May God bless you, Amen.

LUNG INFLAMMATION

Often, we find that irritating substances in our environment, as well as infectious diseases, cause our lungs to become inflamed; this is generally referred to as pneumonia. Our lungs are a very important organ within our body as they allow oxygen to enter the body and carbon dioxide to defuse. Without our lungs, the other organs of the body cannot function therefore protecting our lung health is vital for good health.

To protect our lungs, it is highly important to follow a healthy alkaline diet to restore the body's balance from a cold and sore throat. Exercising is also vital, as well as eating foods rich in antioxidants and avoiding smoking and smokers. Foods rich in antioxidants are broccoli, wild blue berries, spinach, carrots, potatoes, avocadoes, kale, radish, cabbages, sweet potatoes, etc. It is important to note that all foods rich in carotenoids, lutein, lycopene, vitamins and selenium are good antioxidants that help neutralize free radicals from the body.

When contracting a cold or the flu, the nose and throat should be kept clean. This can be done by simply sniffing some warm salt water up the nostril and then blowing it out alternately. This is done by keeping one side of the nostril closed by holding it down meanwhile blowing out through the unobstructed side. Use one teaspoon of salt to one pint of warm water. This can be done regularly up to 2-3 times per day. Salt water may be used to gargle and rinse out the mouth as well if the throat is infected. Take a round teaspoon of golden seal and one-fourth teaspoon of gum myrrh and steep this in one pint of boiling water. Use this the same way as the above, ensuring you gargle very deep and well. It will clean out all the bad germs and impurities in the mouth and throat. If this remedy is repeated often enough, the cold or flu will not go into the lungs.

To ensure that the lung is not seriously inflamed, please take internally one tablespoon of this same mixture of the golden seal and gum myrrh at least 2-3 times a day. A hot footbath is very important to keep the lungs open and healthy. An enema or a herbal laxative is also helpful in clearing the body of toxins. There is another very important part of taking care of our lungs that must not be forgotten. That is WATER. It is necessary to drink large quantities of water to maintain moisture in the lung.

Another way to treat chest congestion/cough is to give the patient a hot fomentation to the chest and back of the lungs. Using a short cold towel, rub between each hot fomentation. This helps the blood to flow more freely, allowing for more relief in the affected area. It is also known that steam moisturizes the stuffy area and provides relief. Patients suffering from chest infections are often advised to go on a liquid diet for 2-3 days and should consume mostly citrus products.

This includes but is not limited to unsweetened lemonade, grapefruit juice, orange juice and pineapple juice. Other fruit juices can also be used if there is a high fever. Use this diet until the temperature returns to its near-normal stage.

While the patient's diet is severely restricted during this time, they will require more nourishment to maintain healthy body weight. During this treatment, the patient may consume strained vegetable broth or soybean milk with whole wheat flakes etc. To speed up the recovery process, some herbs may be brewed as a tonic. These are comfrey, cudweed, ginger and ground ivy.

Many foods are good antibiotics and therefore help relieve inflammation. These foods are garlic, turmeric, onion, carrot, dark leafy greens and chili pepper. These foods are rich in antioxidants. Fruits/juices are also very good as well. Some drinks for the lungs are water, green juice, blueberry juice, ginger beer and pomegranate juice. Take care of your health from your thyroid glands which may lead to pulmonary problems such as the weakening of the respiratory muscles to your lungs by keeping them clean.

3 John v2 says, "Beloved, I wish above all things that thou mayest prosper and be in health even as your soul prospereth."

THE SECRET OF FASTING

It is often said that fasting is God's secret weapon for man. in the book of Matthew, chapter Four, we read that Jesus fasted for 40 days in order to empower himself with the Holy Spirit. It is believed that fasting enables the soul to reveal its true condition through the blessings and guidance of the Holy Spirit. When we fast, we also seek to gain that same empowerment through the blessings of God.

Fasting is not only a holy communication with God, but it is also a way to overcome many types of illnesses as it allows the body to be in an optimal state. There are many different types of fasting that we may choose from. Intermittent fasting is the first we will discuss. This type of fasting allows for eating between cycles of fasting, allowing us to experience amazing health results for the whole being. We also have the full fast, or what we call the water-only fast for a period of days as well as the liquid or juice fast and the Daniel fast, where we do not consume any meat, sweets or bread. When people fast, they slow down the rate of infectious diseases affecting their well-being. Fasting also restores our strength as well as restores the intimacy in our relationship with God. It also helps us develop mastery of self and restore our control of the body. For cellular regeneration, we are encouraged to fast for 1-3 days. During this process, the body eliminates unhealthy and dysfunctional cells and replaces them with newer, healthier cells.

Research has shown that intermittent fasting can help lower high blood pressure, reduce the cholesterol level, and control the blood sugar level. Fasting may help lower the blood glucose level, inhibiting cancer cell growth and regeneration. Ketones are often released during fasting, which may aid patients who have Parkinson's disease by protecting the neurons. This may also aid patients who have dementia and Alzheimer's as well. Intermittent fasting may also aid the body in getting good sleep as it may lower the Orexin-A levels at night, allowing for more rest.

Fasting may also help detox the body and is a perfect way to lose weight. Fasting also enables the body to heal and repair its tissues and cells. Fasting is a GOD-given blessing to all humanity as HE will heal you spiritually and physically. St. Augustine once said fasting is a way for the soul to be cleansed and for the mind to be raised upward to GOD. He stated that fasting will also subject one's flesh to the spirit and will render a contrite and humble heart.

Through fasting, one may gain power over physical desires as it quiets the inner self. Fasting relieves the body from many stresses that encumber it. And while we fast, JUST REMEMBER THAT GOD IS THE CREATOR OF LOVE THAT EMPOWERS THE WHOLE HUMAN RACE. MAY GOD BE WITH YOU ALL, AMEN.

PART TWO

THE HIDDEN SECRET OF FOOD AND HERBS

Millions of people worldwide are struggling to attain and maintain a positive health condition to stay free from all manner of diseases and health complications.

The very first step to achieving a healthy state of being is to maintain an alkaline diet. This allows the body to have a balanced PH, meaning its environment is not too acidic. The body's overall health is built significantly in a more alkaline environment.

In order to attain and maintain this state, we must thoroughly cleanse the body of all harmful toxins and waste matter. This allows all body organs to maintain optical conditioning to carry out their functions. To achieve an alkaline state within the body, we must first start with the blood. Just remember that your life is tied up in the blood. Therefore, the bloodstream must be cleansed of all pathogens and toxins in order for our organs to function properly.

To sustain our life and maintain our growth, food is an essential part of the necessities of life. Hippocrates once said, "Let thy food be thy medicine and thy medicine your food." This emphasizes the importance of nutrition for the functionality of the body and how a healthy body may prevent many illnesses. A good diet is one of our most important tools when fighting diseases.

Often due to financial constraints, the convenience of fast foods, scarcity as well as the distance to organic foods, we allow our diet to become a nemesis to our bodies. Changing our dietary habits must become our priority as we go forward. Remember, a balanced diet does not have to be bland or tasteless, so let's get creative in our kitchens. Let's let this be our resolution going forward to rid ourselves of junk foods, abstain from drinking alcohol and cigarette smoking, sodas (coco cola), energy drinks, etc.

For a healthy life, these organs have to function well. The liver, kidney, lungs, skin, spleen, heart, spine and most of all, the brain—is the king of them all. Here is a list of the hidden secret of the food you are looking for.

GARLIC

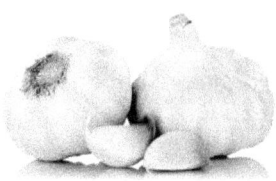

Garlic extracts are filled with antioxidants, antibiotic, and antibacterial properties, allicin which may inhibit the proliferation of bacteria and fungi. Garlic may be used to help fight against high blood pressure, is good for brain health, kidney and liver, and gut health, improves bone health, slows down cancer cells, improves skin and hair, and protects heart health by reversing clogged arteries. Garlic is good for cardiovascular diseases.

GINGER

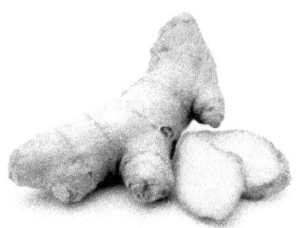

Ginger comes from the underground stem of the ginger plant and is a great spice used in many different dishes around the world. It is packed with antioxidants and has anti-inflammation properties.

It increases the serotonin and dopamine levels in the brain which may reduce inflammation. Ginger offers great help in managing blood sugar levels, fighting stomach ulcers, and relieving gas; great for weight loss while improving the digestive system. It also aids in boosting nutrient absorption, improves breath, relieves pain by relaxing the muscles and soothes migraine. Ginger also greatly boosts the immune system while helping to clear up sinuses. Ginger has wonderful cancer-fighting properties and is very good for the kidney's overall health. This little-known root vegetable (FYI, a stem) helps fight Alzheimer's and dementia in patients, relieves menstrual pain, and is a good remedy for fungal infections while improving overall brain function.

TURMERIC

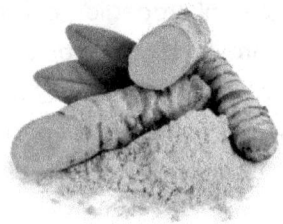

The active property is curcumin. It has anti-inflammatory and antibacterial use and helps to maintain blood sugar levels, weight loss, and relieve clogged arteries. Its active property, curcumin, for centuries has been used in the treatment of depression and anxiety.

Turmeric is also very good in the treatment of scabies. It has anticancer properties, great for liver health, and strengthens our immune system by enhancing our body's antibody responses. Turmeric is also great for overall kidney health, helps to relieve sore throat, and is good for urinary function and prostate health.

Due to its antioxidant and anti-inflammatory properties, turmeric has been used as a supplementary treatment for Inflammatory Bowel Disease (IBD). It is also excellent for brain health as its active property curcumin helps to increase the growth of new neurons in the brain, which may help to fight various cognitive degenerative diseases such as Alzheimer and dementia.

Turmeric's anti-inflammatory and antioxidant properties help boost blood sugar levels in diabetic patients. It is also very good for overall skin health and many more diseases.

Important information to note is that when using turmeric for health purposes, in order to realize its complete potency of it, a pinch of black pepper, which is full of piperine, may be added. Piperine is known to have many pharmacological effects and is an alkaloid that has antioxidant and anticancer properties, to name a few.

KALE

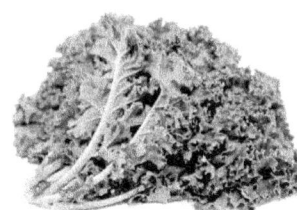

Kale has many health benefits that are of vital importance to the overall well-being of the body. Its properties are:

Kale is rich in vitamins A, C, K and B6, which aids in improving the immune system and good bone health and helps to alleviate and prevent chronic health issues, and aid in brain development. It has antioxidants, anti-inflammatory and antiviral use, and very high beta carotene, which helps the body fight free radicals that damage the cells.

Kale is rich in magnesium which aids in the protection against type 2 diabetes and heart disease. It is a good plant-based source of calcium, a nutrient that is very important for bone health is also high in lutein and zeaxanthin, two powerful carotenoid nutrients that help to protect the eyes.

Kale can help lower the cholesterol level, which may reduce the risk of heart disease and is critical for blood clotting as it is rich in vitamin K.

It helps to fight the formation of cancer at the molecular level as it is full of phytochemicals. Research has shown that kale helps the body fight colon, breast and prostate cancer, to name a few. It is a great source of minerals, as well as a great help for the body to lose weight.

BLUEBERRY

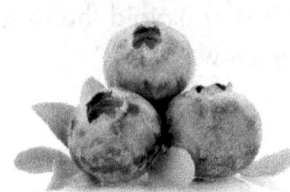

Blueberry is said to boast an impressive nutritional profile that helps the body to boost its immune system and a whole host of other benefits. It is full of fiber and is very tasty while being nutritious. Properties of blueberry:

It reduces blood pressure while protecting the body against aging and wrinkles, as well as maintaining the cholesterol level. Blueberries are filled with flavonoids that help to boost the immune system and prevent memory loss.

Blueberries lower the risk of heart disease and cancer. It helps fight cancer all over the body, such as breast and colon and prostate cancer. It also contains chemicals that are used to stimulate and promote hair growth as well as improve your vision.

Blueberry also aids digestion by preventing constipation and maintaining a healthy digestive tract because of its fibrous content. It is also good for type 2 diabetes as well as boosting brain health. Blueberries are low in calories and very high in nutrients such as vitamins C, K, A, B9, B12 and B6.

Blueberries help to fight against urinary tract infections as well as help to lower muscle damage and lower blood sugar. Blueberries help reduce inflammation in the body because they are rich in antioxidants and reduce damage to the DNA chain.

Blueberries also help to reduce blood clotting and are good for the cardiovascular system overall.

BLACKBERRIES

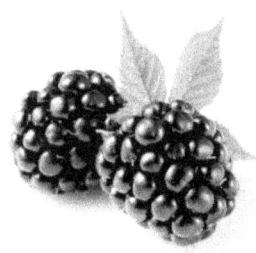

Blackberries are a rich source of anti-cyanins with many anti-inflammatory and anti microbial properties. It contains powerful antioxidants which help to detoxify the body's system. Blackberries are also filled with minerals such as potassium, manganese, magnesium, phosphorus, calcium, insulin, lutein, calories, and vitamins.

Blackberries help to manage type 2 diabetes, reduce high blood sugar levels, as well as good for overall bone health. It is also a good source of brain health as it helps to prevent memory loss from aging.

Blackberries also help in lowering blood pressure and aid in the prevention of Parkinson's disease.

Blackberries fight against urinary tract infections and are very good for lowering cholesterol levels. It lowers the blood sugar level and is very good for your vision. Blackberries can boost your immune system through their phytochemical properties that fight free radicals, which help to reduce the risk of cancer.

RASPBERRIES

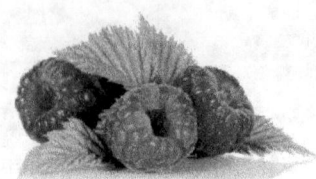

Raspberries have myriad benefits, from helping to prevent heart disease and stroke to lowering blood pressure and sugar to a whole host of other amazing benefits. Its properties are:

Raspberries are high in antioxidants, fiber and vitamins. It has anti-inflammatory and anticancer properties as well as rich minerals such as; manganese, potassium, copper, magnesium, calcium, and zinc.

Raspberries have anthocyanin, which helps reduce oxidative stress to the body, beta carotene, and vitamin C, b6, K, and E. Regular consumption helps lower cholesterol and improves digestive health.

Raspberries are known to significantly boost the immune system as they are rich in antioxidants that help eliminate inflammation. They also have a rich water and fiber content which is helpful to the digestive tract as it helps to prevent constipation and promotes regular bowel movement.

Raspberries are also low in calories and greatly help reduce blood pressure due to their potassium content, which is essential for heart health. It is very good for bone and skin health and improves liver health. Raspberries also aid in weight loss, combat aging, as well as sharpen your brain and improve memory.

STRAWBERRIES

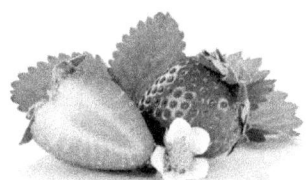

Strawberries are rich in nutrients that are essential for our daily health. It is packed with antioxidants, potassium which is essential for heart health, and other minerals such as manganese and magnesium. Strawberries are also rich in quercetin, ellagic acid, and catechins which have potent antioxidant and anti-inflammatory properties. It is also used to promote bone health, as well as help to protect cardiovascular health.

Strawberries are also used to lower bad cholesterol, have high fiber content, and regulate blood pressure levels. It is also used to prevent type 2 diabetes, improve vision, and help lose weight while keeping wrinkles at bay.

Another important function strawberries provide for the body is restricting inflammation and decreasing cancer cell growth. Strawberries are high in vitamin C as well as trace amounts of vitamin K which are great antioxidants.

BEET ROOT

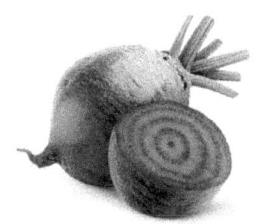

Beets are packed with essential nutrients and are a great source of fiber and other minerals. It is associated with many benefits, such as improved blood flow and blood pressure. Some of its properties are:

Beets have powerful antioxidant and anti-inflammatory properties. It is rich in potassium which supports heart health. It has lycopene; methionine, calcium for bone health; vitamin C and b6. Beets also help maintain a healthy weight, which is good for the digestive system by relieving constipation. It also helps to protect from premature aging as it is good for the skin. It prevents hair loss, is a natural detox agent, improves liver function and improves exercise stamina.

Beets are a good source of purifying blood. It helps to cure arthritis as well as help to lower high blood pressure. Studies have shown that beets lower blood glucose levels and control the body's insulin. It is a great help to diabetics as it allows more sensitivity to insulin.

Beets may also prevent colon, breast and prostate cancer. Numerous studies have shown that beetroot are highly beneficial to patients who undergo chemo as it helps to slow down active tumor in the body due to its active compound, belatin.

Beets are often used as a gout and pigmentation remedy. It is also good for anemia, is a fertility helper, as well as helps in circulation and helps promote good mental health. It is also good for the overall health of the lungs.

Beets are important in promoting brain health. Beets are filled with nitrate oxide, which helps the body's blood vessels constrict and dilate, which helps to improve blood pressure. It is also water-soluble, low in calories and a good fiber source. People that consume a lot of beetroot juice will have a better overall health value in their lifetime.

POMEGRANATE

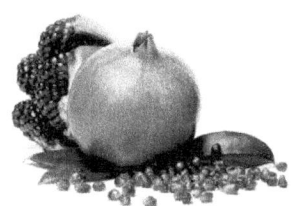

Pomegranate is a sweet, tart fruit that is fun to eat and provides a wide range of health benefits to the body. The properties of pomegranate are:

Antioxidants that help to prevent or delay cell damage. Anti-inflammatory substances, potassium, polyphenols, folate acid, iron, fiber, vitamins A, C, E, K. Pomegranate may be used to help fight and prevent gout due to its citric and malic acid content, which helps to control uric acid levels. It may also be used to lower the risk of prostate, breast and lung cancer, as studies have shown that it hinders the growth of existing cancer cells as well as various other effects.

Pomegranate also helps to fight off Alzheimer's disease as its polyphenols are said to be neuro protective. It reduces inflammation in the microglia, which are specific cells in the brain. It is also good for digestion as it is rich in fiber and relieves arthritis and osteoarthritis pain. Pomegranate is very good for heart disease as it offers abundant benefits for the cardiovascular system, such as blocking triglycerides. This allows for the body's cholesterol level to be lowered as pomegranates reduce plaque buildup in the arteries. It is also good for enhancing sexual performance as it improves blood flow and increases testosterone levels.

Another health benefit of pomegranate is that it helps with diabetes as it aids with reducing insulin resistance in the body. Pomegranates are filled with essential vitamins and are full of nutrition which is helpful to the body. Pomegranate is very good for ulcers as it promotes good gut health due to its active compounds that reduce stomach inflammation and promote healthy bacteria. It also strengthens the immune system by boosting antibody production due to its rich antioxidant properties. Pomegranate helps to strengthen and regenerate bones and helps prevent cartilage damage. Its peel is a good exfoliator that removes dead skin cells and boosts collagen production. They are also useful in helping to prevent cataracts in older adults.

Iron is necessary for many functions in the body to be carried out, such as hemoglobin production. Pomegranates, due to their high vitamin C content, allow the body to absorb and assimilate iron, which may prevent anemia.

Pomegranate is good for weight loss as it prevents triglycerides from being stored in the body as fats. It is rich in vitamin B complex. Overall, pomegranate juice and oil from its seeds are an excellent choice for the body.

CLOVE

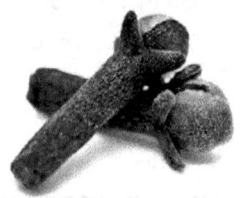

Cloves are one of the spices used in Asia and some parts of the world and have numerous health benefits. It may be found in mostly tropical climates. It comes from *Syzygium aromaticum,* otherwise known as the clove tree. The clove as many health benefits, such as;

Cloves have anticancer properties due to their anti-inflammatory, antibacterial, antiseptic, antimicrobial, antiviral and antioxidant properties. Studies have shown that cloves may be used to inhibit the growth of tumors as well as induce and encourage apoptosis (programmed cell death) of cancer cells. It has been hailed as a potent agent that enhances chemotherapy and is an anti- carcinogenic agent.

Cloves contain eugenol, calcium, and vitamins C and K. It is a very good source for improving digestion as it stimulates enzyme secretions by helping to reduce bloating, gastric irritation and flatulence. Cloves are full of antioxidants which are helpful in reducing inflammation. This helps boost the immune system by fighting bacterial infections thanks to its active compound, eugenol and other compounds. When used with warm water, cloves relieve coughs and colds.

The liver is a very important organ in the body as it breakdown fats, aids in the metabolic processes as well as produces energy for the body to carry out its functions. Clove is a good source for improving and promoting liver function due to its rich anti-oxidative properties. Antioxidants, as we learned previously, are very important in eliminating free radicals from the body. Cloves contain eugenol, which is very important in helping the liver fight liver disease and many other ailments affecting the liver. Cloves also help to prevent gout by eliminating excess uric acid and reducing inflammation. Cloves are high in manganese, eugenol and potassium, an essential mineral that is vital for brain health. The oil made from clove stimulates the circulatory system, reduces stress and anxiety, reduces insomnia, and boosts memory.

The bones provide the body with stability and mobility. It is also responsible for producing the blood cells as well as most of the body's calcium supply. Cloves are one of the more useful spices we regularly consume that may enhance bone health. Studies show that its eugenol and flavonoid compound increases bone density and mineral content. It also improves several of the markers of osteoporosis. Cloves are widely known to promote insulin production as well as aid in keeping blood sugar levels in check. This is because cloves are rich in antioxidants and digestive health benefits that aid with diabetes.

Cloves are also great in the fight against gram-positive and negative bacteria. It also stimulates libido by increasing testosterone, as it has many aphrodisiac properties. Cloves are also good for your skin health. It is a powerful anti-aging ingredient often found in women's cosmetic products. Cloves are said to remove dead skin cells as well as reverse fine lines and wrinkles.

BRUSSELS SPROUT

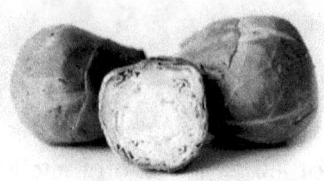

Brussels sprouts are one of the cruciferous vegetables that can be counted on to boost the immune system. It is deemed one of the super foods that are rich in fiber, vitamins and minerals that are essential to the overall health of the body. Brussels sprouts are filled with antioxidants, anti-inflammatory properties, folate acid, minerals (manganese, potassium, copper), and vitamins C, B6, B1, and K. It may reduce cancer cell growth.

Brussels sprouts may also be used to reduce the effects of heart disease. It may be used to reduce inflammation, improve blood circulation, and control blood sugar to prevent diabetes. Brussels sprouts may help to prevent constipation due to the support of probiotic health. It supports bone health while also promoting good skin health. Another important function of Brussels sprout is that it is very good for your brain and nerve health. It is a good energy supply base; it supports your red blood cells. Brussels sprout is a good source of anthocyanin, beta carotene, potassium, magnesium, iron, sulforaphane, anticancer, and vitamins A, B6, C, D, and K. When Brussels sprout is used along with cabbage. It aids in the prevention of bowel problems such as constipation. It aids in the overall health of the colon, lungs, prostate and breast cancer.

CABBAGE

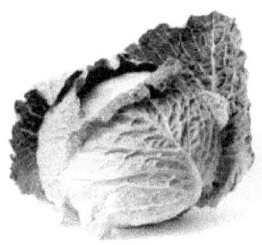

Cabbage is good for the heart as it may help reduce bad cholesterol that may cause plaque buildup in the arteries. Cabbage is beneficial for digestive health, vision, and lowering blood pressure. Eating cabbage regularly has significant benefits for the skin as it has anti-aging properties. It is filled with antioxidants that may reduce the free radicals responsible for damaging skin cells as well as boost collagen production. Like many other cruciferous vegetables, cabbage is good for the removal of toxins from the blood due to the sulforaphane found within it. It also contains glutathione, an antioxidant that aids the liver in its detoxification function.

Cabbage stimulates hair growth due to its vitamin A content and is low in calories and high in carbohydrates which are beneficial for blood sugar management. It also aids in the increase of insulin in the body. Cabbage juice is beneficial for those who are suffering from ulcers as it aids in the healing of the intestinal barrier and lining. Cabbage is also good for pregnant women and vitamin K deficiency.

BROCCOLI

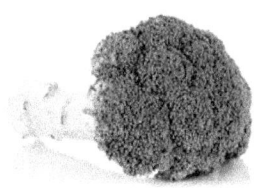

Broccoli is a nutrient-rich vegetable that has many benefits to the overall body. It has many antioxidants, anti-inflammatory, anti-inflammation and anticancer properties.

Broccoli has rich minerals such as copper, iron, zinc, calcium, magnesium, potassium, and manganese. It also has vitamins A and B, and twice the amount of vitamin C than orange and vitamin K. Studies on broccoli show it has the potential to reduce the body's cancer risk. It has a high amount of phytochemicals such as sulforaphane which is a compound that fights against cancer of the colon, prostate, breast, as well as some oral cancers.

Broccoli is very good for heart health as it helps to regulate blood pressure in the body. It works by lowering bad cholesterol, which leads to a healthy heart. Broccoli also helps to keep the blood vessels healthy as it helps prevent damage to them. Broccoli has a rich source of vitamin C, which aids in improving immune function. It functions as an antioxidant which greatly aids the immune system. Broccoli helps to clean up the liver. It is filled with phytochemicals, fiber and antioxidant properties, which support liver health.

Broccoli keeps the bones healthy as it has high levels of vitamin K and calcium minerals which are vital to bone health. A note of caution: If patients have a condition requiring blood thinning medication, broccoli must be taken with caution as it is filled with vitamin K that may inhibit anti-blood coagulating medicine. Please speak to your doctor if you use blood thinners about when it is safe to consume broccoli.

Another important function of broccoli is that it makes the brain healthy. It is filled with brain-healthy antioxidants such as flavonoids and vitamin C. It has compounds that lower the risks of neurodegenerative conditions to improve and maintain memory function. It has important nutrients, such as vitamin B, which helps restore and maintain nerve function.

Broccoli is a food rich in fiber that supports and improves digestion. It is a good source to enhance the growth of good bacteria in the gut, which aids in the prevention of constipation. It also aids in the control of the blood sugar level by lowering elevated blood glucose, which is beneficial to diabetes patients. Broccoli slows down the aging process by reducing oxidative stress on the body's cells. It also helps to maintain dental and eye health.

YAM

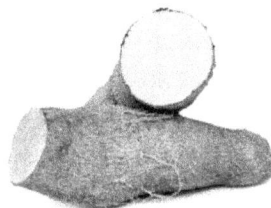

Yams are packed with nutrients and have many properties such as antioxidants, anti-inflammation. These agents/properties may help reduce many chronic illnesses that negatively affect the body. Yams contain beta-carotene, iron, copper, manganese, potassium, folate, thiamine, fibers and plenty of vitamins C and B6. Yam is good for the cardiovascular system due to its anti-inflammatory and antioxidant properties. When eaten on a consistent basis, yams will aid in the lowering of the cholesterol level. It has a rich potassium and fiber nutrient content which aids in heart health. Yams are also good for anti-aging benefits as they protect the skin, hair, and eyes and help with weight loss.

Yams are highly nutritious foods that will improve blood sugar level as it is low in glycemic index content. Yams may also improve insulin sensitivity by reducing insulin resistance due to their high magnesium and fiber content levels. Yams are very good for a healthy nervous system as it aids in the improvement of brain function. Yams are an excellent source that may help to promote fertility and may also aid in the prevention of premature births.

DASHEEN

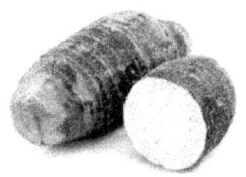

Dasheens are a great source of fiber-rich nutrients-resistant starch that provides the body with a whole host of health benefits.

Dasheens have many properties and benefits, such as; antioxidants, anti-inflammation, manganese, potassium, copper, phosphorous, calcium, and zinc. Dasheens are jam-packed with vitamins A, B1, B2, B6, C, E, and K. It has health benefits such as improved heart and gut health and improved blood sugar management. Due to its rich fiber content, dasheen may aid in improved digestive function and decrease bloating and constipation in the body. It is also filled with good carbohydrates that may aid in the control of the blood sugar level, thus helping to prevent diabetes or reduce its impact on the body. The nutrients in dasheen are also good for skin and eye health.

Another important health benefit of dasheen is that it lowers the cholesterol level, which greatly aids the cardiovascular system. It has polyphenols that protect the body against oxidative stress. The high potassium found in dasheens helps the body break down excess salt in the blood, thus reducing the risk of high blood pressure (IBP). Dasheen is very good for blood pressure as its high level of vitamins B6, C and E may also aid in boosting the immune system through the elimination of free radicals. The potassium found in dasheen is also excellent for increasing blood flow to the brain. It allows for improved cognitive function and neural activities. Dasheen also has a compound called quercetin which is a known cancer-fighting agent. Thus, it may aid in the prevention and elimination of cancer.

PAPAYA

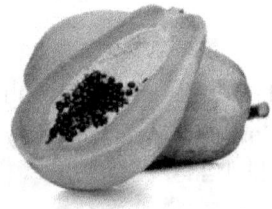

The healing powers of papayas are a well-kept secret that must be unveiled. It is a yellow-orange colored fruit that is often found in tropical areas. It has powerful antioxidants, anticancer, anti-inflammatory, and antibacterial properties. It contains lycopene, papain, bromelain, and minerals such as potassium, copper, iron, and calcium, as well as high levels of vitamins A, C, and E. Papayas also contain vitamins B1, B3, B5, B9 and K. It has been well documented that diets rich in antioxidants may help in reducing the risk of developing heart diseases and strokes. Papayas are fruits that are filled with this compound.

Whether sliced and eaten or used to make a drink, papayas are sweet and enjoyable fruits filled with nutrients. It is good for skin injuries, heart health, improving the digestive system, and reducing inflammation within the body. Papaya juice may aid in lowering cholesterol due to its high antioxidant and vitamin C, A, and E content. The regular consumption of this fruit may aid in regulating blood pressure as well as promote good blood circulation within the arteries. It also increases cortisol output which aids in the reduction of stress, leading to heart problems.

The carotenoids found within papayas help to neutralize free radicals found in the brain, which may lead to Alzheimer and similar diseases. Regular intake of papaya juice may also help protect the eyes from deteriorating as well as aid with chronic sinus issues through its active compound papain. The papain found in papayas is also good for the digestive system by breaking down foods, aiding with constipation and bloating. The fiber content in papayas also aids the colon by binding toxins found from interacting with the healthy cells, thus reducing the risk of colon cancer and other health risks. The enzymes found in papayas aid the body by promoting a balanced and healthy acidic environment, thus reducing the risks of developing ulcers and other inflammations.

Papayas also have anti-aging properties and may aid in the protection of the eyes. It may also provide a boost to the immune system when eaten on a regular basis due to its high vitamin C and beta-carotene level.

PAPAYA LEAF

The leaves of the papaya are often consumed as teas, blended into juices or extracts. Over the years, it has been used to treat infections such as dengue fever as well as to prevent malaria and the like. It has been shown that papaya leaves may be used to treat a variety of bacterial infections. It has all the properties found in the fruit, as well as vitamin B17, which is found in cancer treatment such as chemotherapy. The nutrients found in the papaya leaves are believed to improve the body's immunity. Along with all the papaya fruit's properties, the leaves also contain chymopapain, which breaks down protein.

Papaya leaves carry out the same functions as the fruit. They fight infection in the body, improve digestion, treat stomach ulcers, lower blood sugar, reduce and treat inflammation of the gut, treat skin problems or infections, improve hair growth, and play an integral role in breast cancer treatment.

PAPAYA SEED

The papaya seeds are highly nutritious and provide a wide range of benefits to the body. The seeds of the papaya have powerful antioxidants, the same as the fruit and leaves. They are rich in polyphenols which protect the body against oxidative stress, and flavonoids (anti-inflammatory, antioxidants, antibacterial, and anti-pathogenic) properties. The seeds also contain carpaine, alkaloids and tannins. They have the same minerals and vitamins as the fruit they are taken from.

Papaya seed compounds help maintain cardiovascular health and treat heart problems. It aids in the reduction of inflammation of the joints, kills bacterial and viral infections such as dengue fever and cleanses the kidneys. Some compounds in the seeds may be used to destroy parasites that thrive in the intestine, enhance digestive function, prevent aging, enhance vision, and treat acne breakouts.

Studies have shown that the polyphenols and isothiocyanate found in papaya seeds fight free radicals found in the body to inhibit the development of cancer cells. This prevents or reduces the risk of developing breast, colon, lung, leukemia and prostate cancer growth. Papaya seed may also relieve menstruation pain, relieve and reduce diabetes and heart-related problems, and aid in bowel health due to its laxative properties. Papaya seeds are fiber-rich, thus able to alleviate constipation. It is also able to remove e coli from the intestines.

Papaya seeds may be consumed in the quantity of 15 to 20 per day with a glass of water. It may be used as an excellent cleanse for the liver and colon. A cautionary warning to all men. Papaya seeds may play an adverse effect on men's fertility if consumed in excess amounts. Thus, men who consume the seed must be careful. Overconsumption may cause decreased motility of sperm and low sperm count.

AVOCADO

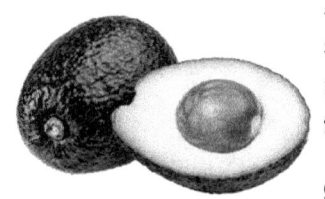

Avocados are known as one of the major superfoods, containing 20 vitamins and minerals. They are classified as fruits though they are part of the vegetable group and are packed with fiber, potassium and a high monounsaturated fat content. It is filled with antioxidants and anti-inflammatory properties. Avocados contain minerals such as manganese, magnesium, potassium, phosphorous, copper, zinc and iron. It has vitamins A, B1, B3, B5, B6, B12, C, D, E, and K. It also contains carotenoids, beta-sitosterol, choline, carotene, lutein, and folate. Daily consumption of avocados may help in weight loss due to their rich fiber content and improved digestive function. They also protect the eyes against UV rays due to their oxidative, lutein and zeaxanthin content.

Avocados are low in carbs, thus are good for people with diabetes as they are on the lower side of the glycemic index. They are packed with oleic acid, fiber, omega 3 and 6 fatty acids, potassium and folate, which are good for heart health. They aid in lowering cholesterol to keep the arteries clear and blood pressure. According to research published in the Journal of American Heart Association, avocados are great for the heart and can reduce the risk of developing heart disease.

Due to its rich fiber content, avocados are essential for a healthy digestive system. It is also rich in monounsaturated fats, which significantly impact the gut microbial population and reduce fecal bile acid concentration. It is also good for bone health due to its rich mineral content, greatly reducing the risk of osteoporosis. Its antioxidants are also good for the health and vitality of the skin as it reduces the risk of premature aging.

Another major health benefit of this fruit is that it is filled with phytochemicals and carotenoids, which studies show may slow down the progression of many cancer cells. These phytochemicals and carotenoids may help in the treatment of leukemia cancer stem cells. Avocados also, due to their strong fiber content and low carb ratio, may help prevent many complications associated with diabetes, such as heart issues and strokes. It may provide improved insulin sensitivity, blood sugar regulation and stability.

The oleic acid and vitamin A, E and C content in avocados may also improve the elasticity or collagen in the skin providing a more youthful look. Its natural oil helps moisturize the skin and relieves inflammation caused by psoriasis and eczema. Its biotin content may encourage the healthy growth of the hair. Studies have shown that the daily consumption of avocados may lead to cognitive improvement and flexibility. It also contains an amino acid called tryptophan, a known mood booster and stabilizer due to its aid in boosting serotonin production. Avocados are also linked to reduced risk of gestational hypertension in pregnant women.

AVOCADO LEAVES

The leaves of the avocado plant provide some of the same benefits as the fruit in a higher concentration. It has more antioxidants and anti-inflammatory properties. It is filled with flavanols, pinene, and polyphenols. They have the same vitamins and minerals as the fruit and seed that are beneficial in improving digestive function, heart and brain health, as well as aid the blood sugar level and liver and kidney health. Avocados are filled with nutrients and may assist persons suffering from anemia, back pain and arthritis. It has analgesic detox properties to cleanse the blood. Avocado leaves provide all the health benefits that may be found in the fruit, just in higher concentrations.

AVOCADO SEED

The seed of the avocado contains soluble fiber and powerful antioxidants, anti-inflammatory, and anticancer properties. It is filled with magnesium, potassium, calcium, and iron minerals. It also contains persin, polyphenols, catechins, protocatechuic, chlorogenic, alkaloids, saponins, pinene, and vitamins A, B1, B6, C, E, and K. The avocado seed may provide inflammation-fighting benefits, aid in the fight against Alzheimer and other neurodegenerative diseases, as well as aiding the digestive system. It may provide help in ridding the body of gastric ulcers and constipation due to its soluble fiber content. It may also aid the body in stabilizing the blood glucose level, thereby aiding the body fight type 2 diabetes, as well as a great aid in losing weight.

Avocado seed is also good for a healthy-looking and feeling skin, fighting pathogens, and improving heart health by lowering the risk of cardiovascular diseases and stroke. They may also aid in cancer-fighting treatments and significantly boost the immune system.

PINEAPPLE

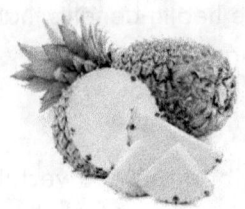

There are many benefits to eating pineapples. Aside from satisfying the taste buds, pineapple provides the body with a significant boost of energy and is known as one of the superfoods that provide us with myriad health benefits. They are packed with antioxidants and have anti-inflammatory and antiviral properties. They contain many minerals, such as manganese, potassium, copper, and calcium. They also contain vitamins A, C, and B6, folate, bromelain, beta carotene, and thiamine. These help to promote healthy bones, digestive aid and heart health. The antioxidants and anti-inflammatory properties found within pineapple juice may help fight and kill cancer cells within the body. These properties may also greatly aid in boosting and promoting the immune system.

Whether eaten sliced or drunk as a juice, pineapples are packed with nutrients that aid in healing and preventing sinus infections, arthritis problem, and inflammation in the body. The bromelain contained within them may aid the digestive tract breakdown of protein. This also helps to eliminate constipation and remove parasites such as e coli from the intestines. Pineapples may also improve eye, hair and skin health due to their lutein and zeaxanthin content.

Pineapple juice is also very excellent for heart health, as it aids in increased blood circulation, reduced blood pressure and reduced plaque buildup from cholesterol. Its active compound, bromain, allows the easy flow of blood, reducing the risk of heart attack or stroke. Pineapple juice is filled with flavonoids, carotenes and polyphenols, which are said to help actively neutralize impurities within the blood. Bromelain may fight against water retention in the body aiding the kidneys to carry out their functions. Pineapple juice may also work to soothe muscle pain, relieve asthma symptoms and eliminate pancreatic insufficiency.

SOURSOP FRUIT

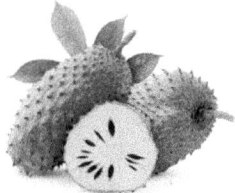

Soursops are said to be filled with antioxidants, anti-inflammatory, antibacterial, antifungal, antiviral, and anti-parasitic properties that may effectively kill off many bacterial infections. It also has anticancer properties and is filled with minerals such as iron, potassium, copper, zinc and calcium. It contains alkaloids, beta carotene, lactones, and vitamin A, B1, B2, C, and E. Soursop juice are rich in fiber and may actively promote weight loss and aid in digestion as it prevents constipation and promotes regularity as well as aid in gastric ulcer treatment. Soursop juice is also believed to fight against free radicals, which damage cells, and fight pathogens to boost the immune system.

It has anticancer properties that may aid in fighting cancer and reduce chemotherapy's side effects. It may aid in the reduction of bad cholesterol and lower blood pressure and uric acid. Patients who suffer from low blood pressure MUST NOT CONSUME SOURSOP. It significantly lowers blood pressure. Soursop extracts were also found to lower blood sugar levels and prevent insulin resistance severely.

Soursop juice may aid in the promotion of bone health, control depression as well as soothe the central nervous system through its active compounds anonaine and asimilobine. Soursop juice may also aid in the treatment of urinary infections by controlling the acidity of the urine. It may also aid in anemia treatment as well as treat some common colds, fever and coughs. The elements contained in soursops are said to be able to aid in reducing the degeneration of the eyes and may prevent cataract development. Soursop juice may also be used in the treatment of eczema and acne. It may also be used for liver health and the gall bladder as it is an alkalinity-producing food thus, it is a good detoxifying agent. Vitamin C and ascorbic acid found in it are also good for skin and hair. You can use the leaves also for the same benefits boiled into tea.

JACKFRUIT

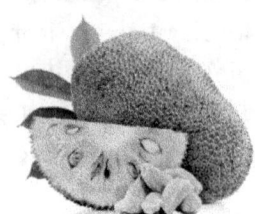

Jackfruit is an exotic tropical fruit known as the world's largest fruit with its fleshy fruit pods. It is sweet and has a distinct taste and flavor that is widely enjoyed in Asia and the Caribbean. It is a fruit filled with potassium and thus may help lower blood pressure and stave off strokes.

Jackfruits also have varied properties such as antioxidants, antimicrobial and anti-inflammatory properties that may ensure better cardiovascular health. It may help to maintain the muscle function in the hearth function as well as a good help to control the cholesterol level.

Jackfruits contain the minerals magnesium, beta carotene, copper, zinc, iron, phosphorous, vitamins; A, B1, B2, B6, C, E, and K, and saponins. Jackfruit is one of the major super foods as it provides so many nutrients for the body. It improves immunity and improves the body's energy supply while being low in sugar. This is why it is believed that jackfruits may help to eliminate type 2 diabetes from the body as it helps with the regulation of blood sugar levels.

Another major benefit of jackfruit is that it may improve digestion and is believed to be very good for bowel health. Its rich fiber content makes it ideal for aiding recovery from ulcers and their prevention while eliminating constipation. It improves blood flow while preventing premature aging and macular degeneration, enhancing vision. It is low in carbs; thus, frequent consumption of this fruit has a major impact on the body's ability to lose weight as well as providing healing benefits to the skin and hair growth function.

The phytonutrients found in jackfruits are believed to help prevent and fight cancer, such as lung, breast, prostate, and skin cancer. For patients on chemotherapy, it may help reduce the risk of developing leukopenia. An important medical note is that for patients suffering from chronic kidney failure, it is recommended that they avoid eating it due to jackfruit's high potassium content. The kidneys help the body remove extra potassium that is not needed. However, patients suffering from this disease should avoid food that is rich in this content.

The rich minerals found in jackfruit are good for strengthening the bones, and thus it is good to eat. It is also very good for improving body muscle and nerve function. Jackfruit extracts are also known to prevent or alleviate the symptoms of asthma. This is due to its rich vitamin C content, which is good for lung function.

JACKFRUIT SEED

The seeds of the Jackfruit are also highly nutritious and must not be wasted as they provide some of the same benefits as the fruit and leaves as well as a few more benefits. Due to its high vitamin B- complex and fiber content, it may greatly aid in lowering the risk of heart disease and other ailments. They provide the same antioxidant, anti-inflammatory and antimicrobial properties as well as minerals as the fruit. Jackfruit seed promotes good blood circulation and may help prevent anemia. Jackfruit seeds are good for your brain function and may be a great detoxifier. Jackfruit seeds are excellent for balancing the electrolyte level.

BREADFRUIT

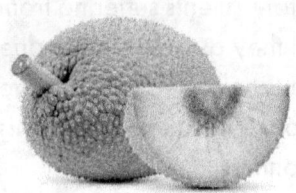

The breadfruit tree produces a round fruit that may be roasted or boiled. It is fiber-rich, which may aid in lowering the risk of diabetes. It is filled with antioxidants which allow the patient to build resistance against many infections that may plague the body. It also boasts anti-inflammatory, antiviral, and anticancer properties. The fruit also contains all the vitamins and minerals that the leaves possess, along with cytotoxins and thiamin. It also aids the heart, kidney, liver, spleen and digestive tract.

Breadfruits help promote collagen in the skin, allowing for the skin's elasticity. It aids in healthy bowel functions by reducing constipation, bloating and cramps. Breadfruit is also very important as it may aid in the reduction of cardiovascular disease in patients. It is good for weight loss, boosting the immune system, and promoting healthy, strong bones. Breadfruit is also a great supplement for brain health. It contains carbs that will keep you full longer and is beneficial for pregnant women. Breadfruit may also be able to reduce certain types of cancer like pancreatic, colon, lung, breast and prostate cancer.

BREADFRUIT LEAVES

Breadfruit leaves are a very powerful healing force, and their health benefits are innumerable. They are rich in compounds such as flavonoids and have high fiber content. The leaves of the breadfruit plant may be used to treat various diseases, such as high blood pressure, diabetes and liver disease. It has many properties, such as anticancer, antioxidant, anti-inflammatory, and antiviral. Breadfruit leaves are filled with polyphenols, potassium, magnesium, iron, copper, calcium, and many vitamins such as A, B1, B2, B3, B6, C, E and K.

When brewed into a tea or herbal concoction, it will reduce inflammation of the legs and feet, reduce water retention from the cells caused by the kidney not functioning well, as well as act as a good detoxifying agent. Breadfruit leaves are good for stress and anxiety, restoring kidney function and repairing the nerves. Another major function of breadfruit leaves is that it is good for hypertension which is a silent and deadly killer. Potassium allows the blood flow with the body to be smooth as it flows through the arteries in which breadfruit leaves are rich. It also regulates the heartbeat and contractions, allowing for normal blood pressure flow. It is filled with omega-3 and six fatty acids, which are highly beneficial for the heart, hair and skin, repairing damaged nerves and improving brain function. The flavonoid content in breadfruit allows it to be effective in treating many illnesses, such as hepatitis, enlargement of the spleen and diabetes. It is effective against gout, kidney stones and the formation of crystals in the joints. Studies have shown that breadfruit leaves are a good remedy for cholesterol as it lowers bad cholesterol and increases good cholesterol. Dosage: Mix one tablespoon of breadfruit powder in 1 liter of water, boiled under low heat until water evaporates halfway. Turn off the stove and refill to one liter, then let sit and cool. Take one cup per day on an empty stomach.

STRONG BACK

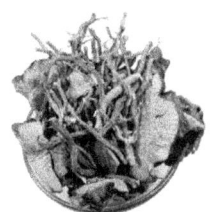

Strong Back contains many pain-relieving properties and is a good remedy for colds and coughs. Drinking it may also aid in better breathing and breast milk production in women. Strong Back is also a very good supplement for the nerves and may aid in the relief of stress from the body. It is also a great remedy to help with improved bowel movements as it aids in ridding the body of parasitic worms. It is great for the entire digestive tract and may promote wound healing and back pain healing. Strong back has also been used to purge and cleanse the blood of impurities. It is also known to aid asthma and bronchial treatments as it is beneficial for respiratory ailments. It may also aid persons suffering from kidney and pulmonary complaints. Taking a dose of 1-2 teaspoons three times daily for a period of 7 days may alleviate most pains and respiratory issues. It may also be used to treat anxiety issues, nerve pain and nervous tension, which may cause migraines. Strong back may alleviate dysentery within the intestines and work as a strong detoxifying agent to cleanse the body from environmental toxins. It may also be a great treatment for anaphylactic shock caused by allergic reactions.

Stress and many other environmental and personal issues may cause many men to experience a low libido or impotence. Strong back may be made into a tonic that improves the energy and stamina in men as well as provide help to alleviate signs of impotence. It may also aid in keeping the microbiome in women in balance. As an external pain remedy, the plant may be soaked in rum or other alcohol and used as a tincture on pain spots as well as boiled into a tonic for oral consumption.

JAMAICAN-SPANISH NEEDLE

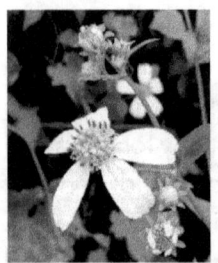

This plant is sometimes referred to as teething bur and is often used to soothe teething babies as it soothes sore gums. Its common name is Biden Alba, Black Jack and Butterfly Needle. This plant carries many benefits that are particularly good for the mucus membrane. It has antibacterial, anti-inflammatory, antimicrobial, antibacterial and anti-malarial properties and benefits. It is neuroprotective and is often used as a nerve tonic and may be used to treat joint pain, colic and stomach ailments as well.

Spanish Needle may also be used as a treatment for diabetics and ailments associated with diabetes, such as heart disease, stroke, kidney failure and loss of sight. It is found that Spanish Needle has hypoglycemic effects as its ethyl acetate and n-butanol compounds were found to have potent anti-diabetic actives. It provides a cleansing effect for liver and kidney detoxification.

Spanish Needle may be used to stop or slow down the effects of angina as it aids in the supply of blood to the heart muscles. Due to its rich fiber, it is believed that it may help reduce bad cholesterol, which frees the arteries from plaque buildup. It aids in lowering blood pressure and the risk of developing hypertension.

Another major health benefit of Spanish needles is that they may aid in hindering cancer cell development. For centuries this plant has been used as an antiseptic used to treat cuts and inflammations. It is also used as a weight loss supplement to rid the body of bloating caused by indigestion and dispel intestinal worms from the body. When made into tea, Spanish Needle calms the stomach and is useful in aiding the menstrual cycle. It relaxes and calms the nerves and provides certain cognitive assistance that aids in mental health.

PERIWINKLE

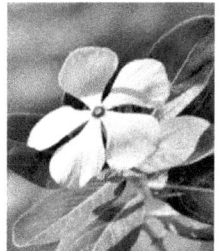

Periwinkle is widely known for its toxicity and comes with a warning; this is a powerful herb that must be used moderately. It has fast-acting healing properties, will and can regulate and control the blood sugar level among many other uses. Periwinkle contains antimicrobial, anticancer, anti-dysenteric, anti-inflammatory and anti-infertility properties. With so many great properties, is it surprising that this herb is able to help in cancer-fighting treatment plans? It is known to fight inflammation which provides a boost to the immune system. It is very useful in fighting diseases such as Hodgkin's disease and Leukemia.

Another great function of periwinkle is that it is an excellent herb to increase blood flow and circulation to the brain. This is an herb that, through the ages, has been used for brain health. It is said to improve metabolic reactions in the brain as well as restore and improve memory and concentration. Patients over the years have reported increased mental productivity. Research also indicates that periwinkle may reduce the premature aging of brain cells and calm the nerves. Studies have also suggested that it may aid patients suffering from neurodegenerative diseases such as Alzheimer's and dementia.

Periwinkle leaves, stem, flowers and root may all be used when concocting herbal teas or remedies (note well, it must be used in small portions, 3-5 leaves per day unless prescribed more). This may be used to lower blood pressure, control hypertension, prevent strokes, and recover from a stroke. it may reduce swelling and inflammation within the body, as well as reduce cholesterol levels.

PERIWRINKLE is also a great tonic for women as well. It may aid in treating abnormal vaginal discharge, promoting the normal flow of the monthly cycle, and promoting the healthy function of the urinary tract. It is also useful in treating sore throat, toothaches, and many skin infections and diseases.

Another benefit of using periwinkle is in the treatment of type 2 diabetes. Some indications suggest that it may reduce the blood sugar level. It is also an excellent bath remedy for inflamed eyes. It may be used in treating several cancers such as breast cancer, removing piles from the body, and treating asthma and tuberculosis. MAY GOD BLESS YOU ALL, AMEN

LANTANA CAMARA

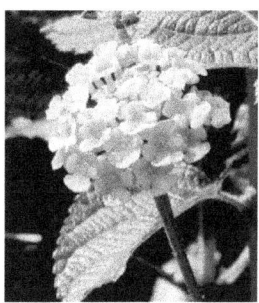

Lantana is a God-given plant to man for the empowerment and healing of the human body. This medicinal plant may be used to heal the body from many different illnesses and diseases. Lantana Camara is a nutrient-dense herb that is jam-packed with medicinal properties such as antioxidants, anti-inflammatory, antifungal, and antimicrobials. It contains anticancer properties and is nematocidal. It may be used to treat disorders of the skin, bilious fevers and colds, as well as digestive and respiratory problems.

Drinking lantana as a tea or herbal tonic may help to remove toxins from the body and promote wound healing. It is a blood purifier that enables the regulation of the platelets in the body and helps boost hemoglobin production in the body. The flower of this plant is often used to treat conditions ranging from dermatitis, eczema, chicken pox, measles, insect bites and swellings, as well as ulcers, tumors, hemoptysis and pulmonary tuberculosis.

This plant has been used to treat various illnesses, and treatments may differ based on geographical location. Studies have shown, however, that its leaves provide an alkaloid fraction that may be used to reduce hypertension in patients as well as asthma and fevers. Its roots are also rich in oleanolic acid and verbascoside, a protein that may aid in cancer therapy.

Patients suffering from digestive complaints such as ulcers have seen significant improvement in their ailment as the plant regulates gastric PH in the stomach. Its only ethyl acetate is effective against most bacteria, especially those that affect the intestines. This amazing herb may also be used to reduce bloating, indigestion and diarrhea. A cautionary note, the LANTANA CAMARA UNRIPED SEEDS ARE TOXIC TO HUMANS AND OTHER ANIMALS.

When made into a poultice to use externally, due to its antiseptic and antimicrobial qualities, it may treat most skin infections or diseases. It may also be used to treat bone and joint complaints and is also a natural pain remedy. The leaves are jam-packed with flavonoids and enzymes that eliminate free radicals that harm the cells of the body. It is a natural detox for the liver and blood.

STINGING NETTLE

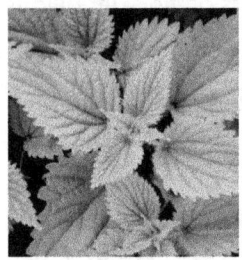

This is an herb that has been used for centuries to treat pain. It has many health benefits that make it one of nature's perfect herbs. It is anti-inflammatory, antibacterial and has a rich source of antioxidants. It is filled with flavonoids and packed with minerals such as; potassium, magnesium, silica, calcium, boron and iron. It has many vitamins, such as; vitamins A, B, C, D, E and K. Stinging Nettle also has folic acid, lutein, and carotenoids. The powerful antioxidants found in the nettle leaves will boost the immune system and protect it from free radicals that damage the cells, thus strengthening the body's immunity. It is a great detox and may remove inflammation from the body.

This herb's high iron and other mineral content and antimicrobial properties make it great for building and cleansing the blood. It is a great detox for both the liver and the kidneys. This may reduce the risk of kidney and liver disorders. Stinging Nettle contains compounds that relax the heart by reducing the force of contraction and thus lowering the pressure. Patients, who suffer from low blood pressure, should not consume this herb. It improves the body's blood circulation, and its beta-sisterol content helps lower cholesterol, thus reducing plaque buildup in the arteries. It is a nourishing and revitalizing herb that re-energizes the body.

Stinging Nettle makes a great tea or tonic and is beneficial for urinary complaints and prostate health, and is a very good treatment for the skin. It is also a wonderful tonic for the digestive system due to its antioxidants and anti-inflammatory content. It reduces the symptoms of acid reflux, bloating, nausea and excess gas, as well as removing parasites from the intestines. It is a good source of calcium and other minerals that are helpful in bone-building and strengthening. It is a great treatment for joint and muscle pain, such as osteoarthritis and osteoporosis.

Another benefit of Stinging Nettles is that it is a great tonic for coughs, sneezing, hay fever and asthma. It removes phlegm from both the lungs and the stomach. The entire plant is a great medicine that may aid in healing many ailments that plague the body. It aids in sleeping, menstrual issues, and premature aging of the skin. It also aids the body in creating a stable balance by calming the nerves and removing tension and stress. The leaves or root may be made into a tincture which may be used topically and internally. It can be used to treat seasonal allergies and fibroids as well as hormone imbalance.

The nettle leaf is a very powerful remedy for type 2 diabetes as it may lower blood sugar as well as aid in diabetic complications such as heart attacks and strokes.

As we heal and nourish the body, let us remember that GOD said that He has given man every herb that yields seed which is on the face of all the earth and every tree whose fruit yields seed for food and health. May God keep you and bless you always, amen.

PART THREE

CLEANSING THE BODY

Cascara Sagrada cause muscle contractions in the intestines that help move stool through the bowels while stimulating liver and secretory functions. The bark of the plant has a laxative effect.

Rhubarb Root is rich in antioxidants and has antibacterial and anti-inflammatory properties. It is highly effective as a laxative and aid in the improvement of the health of the digestive tract through its detoxing effects. It cleanses the body of heavy metals and kills harmful bacteria.

Prodigiosa is an herb that supports healthy kidney function. It stimulates pancreatic juice secretion, reduces blood sugar levels and motivates fat digestion in the gallbladder while improving stomach digestion. It also promotes immune system function.

Burdock Root is known as a powerhouse of antioxidants such as quercetin that have anti-inflammatory effects. It cleanses the liver and lymphatic system by eliminating toxins through the skin and colon. It aids in the filtering of impurities through the bloodstream, controls the blood sugar content, and aids in the prevention of heart disease.

Chaparral cleanses the lymphatic system and removes stress from the liver, supporting its gallbladder function. It also clears heavy metals from the blood and helps in the treatment of diabetes. It is a great pain reliever as well as removing free radicals from the cells.

Dandelion leaves act as a diuretic and has antioxidant properties. It cleanses the kidney, gallbladder, and blood, dissolves kidney stones, removes toxins, and improves blood flow.

Elderberries are jam-packed with antioxidants and vitamins that aid in boosting the immune system. In folk remedies, elderberries are used to remove mucus from the upper respiratory system by treating colds and flu. It is often used to treat kidney complaints and increases urine flow.

Guaco has antibacterial effects that aid in cleansing the blood and skin by promoting perspiration. It reduces inflammation, increases urination and promotes healthy respiratory function. It is also high in iron, strengthens the immune system and may act as a natural blood thinner.

Eucalyptus is a very popular herb found in cough syrups, hair and skin treatment lotions and oils and used as a vapor bath. It is often used to cleanse the skin through steaming/sauna treatments, moisturizing oils, soothe sore throats and treat bronchial or respiratory complaints.

Mullein helps cleanse the lungs by removing mucus. It is a great respiratory tonic that helps open the lungs and soothes coughs and irritations. It helps to open the lungs and soothes coughs and irritations. It creates an anti-inflammatory coating over mucus membranes not just in the respiratory tract but also in the intestines as well.

REVITALIZING HERB

Revitalizing herbs or ayurvedic allows the body to have a boost of vitality and energy through improved digestion. The digestive system is very important for the overall health of the body. Therefore, it is vital to ensure its optimal condition.

Contribo [Duck Flower Vine] helps the body increase energy, appetite, and digestion while promoting good circulation and improving the immune system. It helps the body alleviate constipation, gastritis, remove parasites from the intestines thus promoting good gut health and regulating the menstrual cycle.

Cordoncillo Negro is often used to heal wounds, stop bleeding and vomiting, rid the body of indigestion, kills germs, as well as expelling gas and bacteria. It also helps the body rid itself of some viruses and bacteria reduce mucus inflammation, treat diseases such as gonorrhea, syphilis and other STI's. It is also used to prevent the development of kidney stones and protect the liver.

KALAWALLA

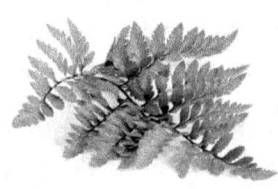

The promotion of harmony and balance is vital to the body's functioning, especially the immune system. Kalawalla is another herb that is a known blood purifier. It is said to provide balance within our bodies by helping to modulate T- cell actives. It is often referred to as an alkaline herb, as it aids in detoxing the body while providing support to the immune system.

Kalawalla is also said to boost and calm the body, thus aiding with fatigue, clearing up bladder problems, protecting the cells within the brain, and reducing inflammation. It is used to treat conditions such as psoriasis, vitiligo, dermatitis and multiple sclerosis. It is also used as a very powerful purge for the body. Reports have shown that kalawalla may also be used to treat auto-immune disorders such as lupus. It also reduces the threat of overacting cells attacking other cells and tissues within the body.

Kalawalla is filled with antioxidants that fight free radicals, natural sun-blocking agents that protect the skin, anti-inflammatory agents that may help fight against cancer, and immune system modulators.

SARSAPARILLA ROOT

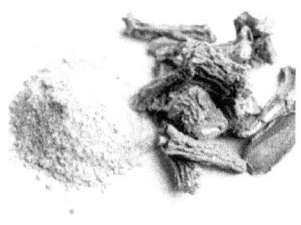

For ages, people have used sarsaparilla root to cure many ailments related to pain. Its phytochemicals have anticancer, anti-inflammatory and antimicrobial benefits. It has been used to heal the pain in the joints, such as arthritis as well as skin conditions, such as psoriasis. Due to its blood-purifying effects, sarsaparilla has been used to treat leprosy, syphilis and herpes.

Sarsaparilla is also one of the best sources of iron. It also contains copper, magnesium, zinc and vitamins A and D. It has a high concentration of saponins as well as natural steroids, which aid in reducing the spread of cancerous cells by inhibiting their multiplication ability. Sarsaparilla root is also known to improve sexual health by improving blood flow.

Another function of the sarsaparilla root is its support for kidney healthy. It is filled with saponins which are known to bind endotoxins and remove them from the body. It is a great detoxing agent that is filled with antioxidant properties.

IRISH MOSS [SEA MOSS]

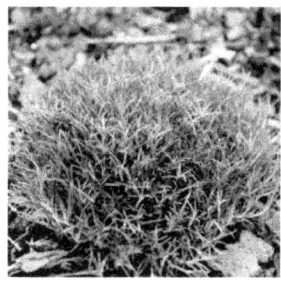

This is a source of nutrient-rich fiber that is vital to maintaining bowel health. Sea moss is also known as a mood booster and a stamina enabler which is particularly good for men as it may reduce the risk of erectile dysfunction. It contains 92 of the 102 minerals the body needs, including Zinc, Magnesium, Iodine, Bromine, Calcium, Iron, Phosphorus, Potassium, and selenium.

Due to its rich content, Irish Moss may help the body control its cholesterol and blood sugar levels. The use of sea moss has been shown to boost the immune system and promotes thyroid and digestive functions. It has antimicrobial, antioxidant and antiviral properties. It is also good for promoting healthy skin. Research has shown that Irish moss may help patients with Parkinson's and other degenerative diseases.

Another benefit of consuming Irish Moss is that it is a rich source of omega-3 fatty acids, magnesium and potassium, which is beneficial for heart health. Studies show that it may be used to regulate blood pressure and lower cholesterol levels. Sea mosses are filled with anti-inflammatory properties that lower the risk of heart disease.

GRANADILLA FRUIT

This fruit contains many antioxidants, anticancer, and anti-inflammatory properties that help to combat free radicals in the body. It is also rich in minerals such as potassium, calcium, phosphorus, and iron; vitamins A, B1, B2, C, and K.

Granadilla fruit has many benefits for the body, such as boosting the immune system and supporting digestive health. When consumed, this fruit is a great remedy for promoting healthy heart function by removing excess cholesterol from the body. It may also help to improve the patient's blood pressure levels.

Granadilla fruit can also help to regulate the blood sugar level due to its low glycemic index. It may also help to improve the body's sensitivity to insulin. The eyes are the lamp of the body; if they are healthy, they provide light to our being. Granadilla has great benefits in improving vision. It is filled with vitamins A, C and flavonoids, which prevents the cells in the eyes from deteriorating due to free radicals, which damages them.

Granadilla is said to be the perfect fruit to reduce inflammation in the body. This is a valuable fruit to strengthen the bone by enhancing its mineral density. Studies have shown that it may help relieve pain that is caused by osteoporosis and osteoarthritis. Another benefit that this fruit provides is antioxidant properties that aid with sleeping and help the body reduce weight.

The pulp in this delicious fruit is rich in fiber, which helps to regulate the digestive system to prevent constipation and other bowel disorders, especially in babies or toddlers. In addition, granadilla fruit may help in the case of diarrhea. It is a soluble fiber that is very powerful and important for the intestinal tract as it may aid in fighting hyperacidity and gastritis ulcers. Granadilla may also aid in relieving coughs, slowdown fevers, etc.

MIMOSA PUDICA

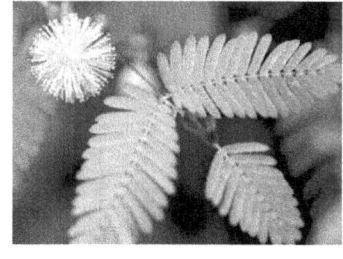

The entire plant is used in herbal tonics to treat many different complaints within the body. It has anti-inflammatory and antimicrobial properties. It may aid fertility treatments and stimulates the promotion of hair growth. It may be used in memory and anxiety treatments by supporting the body's stress response as well as treating hemorrhoids and urinary infections.